This journal belongs to:

_____

_____

"Yesterday is history. Tomorrow is a mystery but today is a gift. That's why they call it the present."

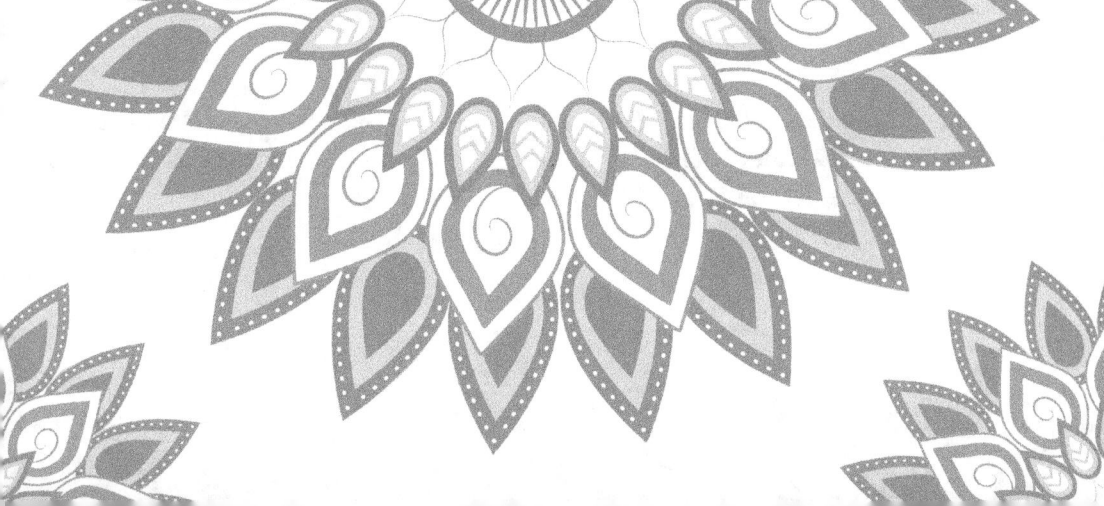

INTRODUCTION

Gratitude—a state of thankfulness—is not a new concept. Ancient texts and scriptures highlight the importance of this unique human emotion in contributing to the richness of our communities, families and inner lives. As Plato pointed out over 2,000 years ago:

"A grateful mind is a great mind, which eventually attracts itself to great things."

In the past 20 years, scientists and psychologists have really buckled down to examine the measurable scientific benefits of gratitude. What they've discovered will change your life. It turns out, feeling grateful isn't just a self-help cliché. The practice of gratitude produces myriad mind-blowing benefits that extend from our psychological to physiological well-being.

Gratefulness is a great tool to enhance your life. Daily gratitude is like medicine for the heart and soul, bringing more and more happiness and wellbeing. Even if you are going through hardship, you can find things to be grateful for, and practicing this will transform your life.

Studies have shown that being thankful can help people feel more positive, relish good experiences, improve their health and build strong relationships with others. It's no secret that our children demonstrate a more positive attitude when practicing thankfulness with their teachers.

To experience the benefits of gratitude, we must practice gratefulness regularly because it doesn't come automatically for most of us. So, if you want to feel gratitude, you must know how to practice gratitude and you must work at it.

How to practice gratitude?

#1 — 30-second morning contemplation with gratitude

Morning contemplation is a great way to develop a habit of daily gratitude. When you first wake up each morning, before you do anything, for at least 30 seconds do this morning contemplation:

- Remind yourself how lucky you are.
- Don't wait to see how you feel that morning, because you're not going to feel good—you're going to feel groggy and tired!
- Just decide that "I'm going to give it everything I've got, to make this day a beautiful day. I'm going to be kind to everyone I meet. I'm going to be gentle and sweet to everyone, even if they hate me. I love my life and I look forward to today."

Every day, before you get out of bed, remind yourself like this. It's a great way to start the day, to protect against the 'weeds' of negative thoughts.

#2 — Switch off your mind

Gratefulness is of the heart, so anything that helps to switch off your mind will tap into the gratefulness of your heart.

Practice meditation and mindfulness so you can be in the present moment, which is exactly where the heart is. When you are in the heart, gratitude will arise naturally. And not only that—living in the present moment will actually benefit every aspect of your life, from health to relationships to success in business.

If you aren't able to control your mind, your thoughts will tell you that, "Oh, I've got nothing worth living for." That's one thought, and then it triggers another thought, "I've got no one around me, I'm lonely." And then another thought, "I'm not sure I can pay the rent this week." There is just one thought after another, and before you know it your daily gratitude practice is out the window.

So switching off your mind is critical in learning how to practice gratitude.

If you'd like help with your meditation practice, try these healing guided meditations with beautiful nature sounds and energy healing infusions.

#3 — Mealtime gratitude practice

Try practicing gratitude at mealtimes. This is easier when you are eating alone or eating with someone who wants to do the same.

Here's how to practice gratitude at mealtimes: just notice things to be thankful for as you eat. It's that easy!

You might be grateful for the taste of the food and the nutritious ingredients you see in the meal. You can feel gratitude for the sun and the earth that provided the food, and the many people involved in the growing and transporting of the food.

Then you might notice the sound of a bird or a dog in the background, and you can feel grateful for animals. You can be mindful of the people you are with or the people you are not with, and you can feel grateful for them, for how they love you or how they challenge you.

The possibilities are endless for how to practice gratitude in this way and it's a great way to develop a habit of daily gratitude.

#4 – Practice kindness and selflessness

When you are kind and giving to others this connects you with your heart, that fountain of gratefulness. Nobody escapes challenges in life, but as long as there is love in our heart the challenges become a delight to encounter and gratefulness can arise.

So, the fourth tip for how to practice gratitude is to practice kindness and selflessness, or to cultivate love. This is perhaps the most powerful spiritual practice you can do, as well as being the easiest.

When we serve others, it awakens the remembrance of our true nature—which is love and compassion. When we help others selflessly, we begin to lose our ego. We dwell more within the heart and less in the mind and thoughts.

Do kind deeds for others whenever the opportunity arises. The kind deeds don't need to be grand but can be as simple as standing on a bus to let an elderly person take a seat, helping a stranger carry their shopping, or interacting kindly with the staff at the supermarket. This then becomes a daily gratitude practice, bringing joy to yourself and others.

#5 – Find inspiration

To progress in any field, you need inspiration. If progress is a car, then inspiration is the wheels. Without the wheels, the car is not going to move forward. So if you're struggling with daily gratitude, find inspiration that makes you feel that life is beautiful.

We are like sponges—whatever we witness, we soak in, and that will become our experience. Try to witness kindness and compassion and love in action. Spend time with people who are happy and grateful and spend time in places that nurture your spirit.

Watch movies or documentaries that show people who are innocent, heroic, honest, honorable, peaceful and loving. Read inspiring quotes and read blogs about love, peace and overcoming challenges. Learn how to connect with your inherent divine power.

All these things will inspire your heart and encourage feelings of gratefulness to arise.

How to stay grateful on a regular basis?

- **Appreciate the little things in life:**

Your life is already filled with friends and family who love and care about you. Forget about the material things you don't have and instead appreciate every single relationship you have and each positive interactive you encounter each day. It doesn't matter how big or small these things are.

- **Say 'Thank you':**

Sometimes we forget to be thankful for the people that are the closest to us. We assume they already know how much we appreciate them. Tell you dad, mom, siblings or friends how thankful you are for them to show them your gratitude.

- **Create a workout routine:**

Did you know that regular exercise can help clear your mind and reduce stress? That's right! Working out not only helps improve your physical health, but will also support your mental wellbeing. Add exercising to your weekly routine and see for yourself!

- **Keep a gratitude journal:**

Jot down all your positive thoughts. Take 5 minutes every night to think about one thing you are thankful for and write it in your gratitude journal. At the end of the week you'll realize that the positives outweigh any negatives.
There's no wrong way to keep a gratitude journal, but here are some general ideas as you get started.
Write down up to five things for which you feel grateful. The physical record is important—don't just do this exercise in your head. The things you list can be relatively small in importance ("The tasty sandwich I had for lunch today.") or relatively large ("My sister gave birth to a healthy baby boy."). The goal of the exercise is to remember a good event, experience, person, or thing in your life—then enjoy the good emotions that come with it.

- **Close each day with gratitude:**

Here is my closing for today: "I'm so grateful that you tuned in to this gratitude practice, and I appreciate your time, your effort, and your energy to be present, awake, and alive to your precious life. "

"*Gratitude is the fairest blossom that springs from the soul*"

Date __/__/__

AM ☀ **I'm grateful for...**

1. _____
2. _____
3. _____
4. _____
5. _____

My potential to succeed is infinite.

PM ☾ **Small victories I had today....**

1. _____
2. _____
3. _____
4. _____

"The root of joy is gratefulness."

Date __/__/__

AM ☀ I'm grateful for...

1. _____
2. _____
3. _____
4. _____
5. _____

Today, I will walk through my fears.

PM ☾ Things I did for myself today....

1. _____
2. _____
3. _____
4. _____

"Wear gratitude like a cloak and it will feed every corner of your life"

Date __/__/__

AM ☀ I'm grateful for...

1. _____
2. _____
3. _____
4. _____
5. _____

I am proud of my own success.

PM ☾ People I'm grateful for today....

1. _____
2. _____
3. _____
4. _____

"It is impossible to feel grateful and depressed in the same moment."

Date __/__/__

AM ☀ I'm grateful for...

1. _____
2. _____
3. _____
4. _____
5. _____

I celebrate my individuality.

PM ☾ 3 Amazing things that happened today....

1. _____
2. _____
3. _____
4. _____

"A moment of gratitude makes a difference in your attitudde"

Date __/__/__

☀ AM **I'm grateful for...**

1. _____
2. _____
3. _____
4. _____
5. _____

I am my own superhero.

☾ PM **How could I have made today even better....**

1. _____
2. _____
3. _____
4. _____

"Things turn out best for people who make the best of the way things turn out."

Date __/__/__

AM ☀ **I'm grateful for...**

1. _____
2. _____
3. _____
4. _____
5. _____

I am free to be myself.

PM ☾ **Small victories I had today....**

1. _____
2. _____
3. _____
4. _____

"Start each day with a positive thought and a grateful heart"

Date __/__/__

AM ☀ I'm grateful for...

1. _____
2. _____
3. _____
4. _____
5. _____

I trust myself.

PM ☾ Things I did for myself today....

1. _____
2. _____
3. _____
4. _____

"Learn to be thankful for what you already have, while you pursue all that you want"

Date __/__/__

AM ☀ **I'm grateful for...**

1. _____
2. _____
3. _____
4. _____
5. _____

I am enough.

PM ☾ **People I'm grateful for today....**

1. _____
2. _____
3. _____
4. _____

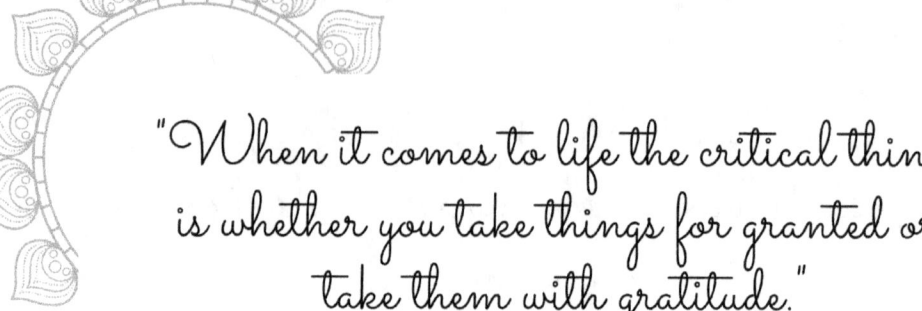

"When it comes to life the critical thing is whether you take things for granted or take them with gratitude."

Date __/__/__

AM ☀ **I'm grateful for...**

1. _____
2. _____
3. _____
4. _____
5. _____

I am whole.

PM ☾ **3 Amazing things that happened today....**

1. _____
2. _____
3. _____
4. _____

"Gratitude unlocks the fullness of life. It turns what we have into enough, and more.."

Date __/__/__

AM ☼ **I'm grateful for...**

1. _____
2. _____
3. _____
4. _____
5. _____

I live each day to the fullest.

PM ☾ **How could I have made today even better....**

1. _____
2. _____
3. _____
4. _____

"No duty is more urgent than giving thanks"

Date __/__/__

AM ☀ I'm grateful for...

1. _____
2. _____
3. _____
4. _____
5. _____

My potential to succeed is infinite.

PM ☾ Small victories I had today....

1. _____
2. _____
3. _____
4. _____

"Enjoy the little things, for one day you may look back and realize they were ....the big things."

Date __/__/__

AM ☀ **I'm grateful for...**

1. _____

2. _____

3. _____

4. _____

5. _____

I take pride in the progress I make each day.

PM ☾ **Things I did for myself today....**

1. _____

2. _____

3. _____

4. _____

"The invariable mark of wisdom is to seek the miraculous in the common"

Date __/__/__

AM ☀ I'm grateful for...

1. _____
2. _____
3. _____
4. _____
5. _____

I am proud of myself and all that I have accomplished.

PM ☾ People I'm grateful for today....

1. _____
2. _____
3. _____
4. _____

"Through the eyes of gratitude, everything is a miracle."

Date __/__/__

AM ☼ **I'm grateful for...**

1. _____
2. _____
3. _____
4. _____
5. _____

I respect and treat myself with kindness and love.

PM ☾ **3 Amazing things that happened today....**

1. _____
2. _____
3. _____
4. _____

"The struggle ends when the gratitude begins."

Date __/__/__

AM ☀ **I'm grateful for...**

1. _____
2. _____
3. _____
4. _____
5. _____

People like me, and I feel good about myself.

PM ☾ **How could I have made today even better....**

1. _____
2. _____
3. _____
4. _____

"Feeling gratitude and not expressing it is like wrapping a present and not giving it.."

Date __/__/__

AM ☀ **I'm grateful for...**

1. _____
2. _____
3. _____
4. _____
5. _____

The world is a better place with me in it.

PM ☾ **Small victories I had today....**

1. _____
2. _____
3. _____
4. _____

"I would maintain that thanks are the highest form of thought and that gratitude is happiness doubled by wonder."

Date __/__/__

AM ☀ **I'm grateful for...**

1. _____
2. _____
3. _____
4. _____
5. _____

I go for goals with passion and pride.

PM ☾ **Things I did for myself today....**

1. _____
2. _____
3. _____
4. _____

"If you count all your assets, you always show a profit."

Date __/__/__

AM ☀ **I'm grateful for...**

1. _____
2. _____
3. _____
4. _____
5. _____

I am never a burden.

PM ☾ **People I'm grateful for today....**

1. _____
2. _____
3. _____
4. _____

"Gratitude is the ability to experience life as a gift. It liberates us from the prison of self-preoccupation."

Date __/__/__

AM ☀ **I'm grateful for...**

1. _____
2. _____
3. _____
4. _____
5. _____

I am worthy of greatness.

PM ☾ **3 Amazing things that happened today....**

1. _____
2. _____
3. _____
4. _____

"If you want to turn your life around, try thankfulness. It will change your life mightily."

Date __/__/__

AM ☀ I'm grateful for...

1. _____
2. _____
3. _____
4. _____
5. _____

I am smart, capable and valuable.

PM ☾ How could I have made today even better....

1. _____
2. _____
3. _____
4. _____

"Gratitude and attitude are not challenges; they are choices."

Date __/__/__

AM ☀ I'm grateful for...

1. _____
2. _____
3. _____
4. _____
5. _____

I am at peace with myself.

PM ☾ Small victories I had today....

1. _____
2. _____
3. _____
4. _____

> *"When I started counting my blessings, my whole life turned around."*

Date __/__/__

AM ☀ I'm grateful for...

1. _____
2. _____
3. _____
4. _____
5. _____

I accept myself as I am.

PM ☾ Things I did for myself today....

1. _____
2. _____
3. _____
4. _____

"Gratitude is a currency that we can mint for ourselves, and spend without fear of bankruptcy."

Date __/__/__

AM ☀ I'm grateful for...

1. _____
2. _____
3. _____
4. _____
5. _____

I am unique in my own wonderful way.

PM ☾ People I'm grateful for today....

1. _____
2. _____
3. _____
4. _____

"The deepest craving of human nature is the need to be appreciated."

Date __/__/__

AM ☀ I'm grateful for...

1. _____
2. _____
3. _____
4. _____
5. _____

I love myself.

PM ☾ 3 Amazing things that happened today....

1. _____
2. _____
3. _____
4. _____

"One can never pay in gratitude; one can only pay 'in kind' somewhere else in life."

Date __/__/__

AM ☀ I'm grateful for...

1. _____
2. _____
3. _____
4. _____
5. _____

I am focused, persistent and will never quit.

PM ☾ How could I have made today even better....

1. _____
2. _____
3. _____
4. _____

"We can only be said to be alive in those moments when our hearts are conscious of our treasures."

Date __/__/__

AM ☀ **I'm grateful for...**

1. _____
2. _____
3. _____
4. _____
5. _____

I am in charge of my own happiness.

PM ☾ **Small victories I had today....**

1. _____
2. _____
3. _____
4. _____

"Gratitude also opens your eyes to the limitless potential of the universe, while dissatisfaction closes your eyes to it."

Date __/__/__

AM ☀ I'm grateful for...

1. _____
2. _____
3. _____
4. _____
5. _____

I have the power to create change.

PM ☾ Things I did for myself today....

1. _____
2. _____
3. _____
4. _____

"Gratitude is more of a compliment to yourself than someone else.."

Date __/__/__

AM ☀ I'm grateful for...

1. _____
2. _____
3. _____
4. _____
5. _____

I take pride in my achievements.

PM ☾ People I'm grateful for today....

1. _____
2. _____
3. _____
4. _____

"Keep your eyes open and try to catch people in your company doing something right, then praise them for it"

Date __/__/__

AM ☀ I'm grateful for...

1. _____
2. _____
3. _____
4. _____
5. _____

I have courage and confidence.

PM ☾ 3 Amazing things that happened today....

1. _____
2. _____
3. _____
4. _____

"In life, one has a choice to take one of two paths: to wait for some special day - or to celebrate each special day.."

Date __/__/__

AM ☀ **I'm grateful for...**

1. _____
2. _____
3. _____
4. _____
5. _____

I can get through anything.

PM ☾ **How could I have made today even better....**

1. _____
2. _____
3. _____
4. _____

"Thankfulness is the quickest path to joy."

Date __/__/__

AM ☀ I'm grateful for...

1. _____
2. _____
3. _____
4. _____
5. _____

I don't need to be perfect.

PM ☾ Small victories I had today....

1. _____
2. _____
3. _____
4. _____

"If the only prayer you said in your whole life was "thank you" that would suffice."

Date __/__/__

AM ☀ I'm grateful for...

1. _____
2. _____
3. _____
4. _____
5. _____

I am an amazing person.

PM ☾ Things I did for myself today....

1. _____
2. _____
3. _____
4. _____

"*Gratitude is riches.
Complaint is poverty..*"

Date __/__/__

AM ☼ I'm grateful for...

1. _____
2. _____
3. _____
4. _____
5. _____

I love myself.

PM ☾ People I'm grateful for today....

1. _____
2. _____
3. _____
4. _____

"Stop now. Enjoy the moment.
It's now or never.."

Date __/__/__

AM ☀ I'm grateful for...

1. _____
2. _____
3. _____
4. _____
5. _____

I can do anything.

PM ☾ 3 Amazing things that happened today....

1. _____
2. _____
3. _____
4. _____

"Give thanks for a little and you will find a lot."

Date __/__/__

AM ☀ I'm grateful for...

1. _____
2. _____
3. _____
4. _____
5. _____

I can make a difference.

PM ☾ How could I have made today even better....

1. _____
2. _____
3. _____
4. _____

"Gratitude is what you feel when you want what you already have."

Date __/__/__

AM ☼ **I'm grateful for...**

1. _____
2. _____
3. _____
4. _____
5. _____

I am in charge of my life.

PM ☾ **Small victories I had today....**

1. _____
2. _____
3. _____
4. _____

*"Appreciation is a wonderful thing.
It makes what is excellent in others
belong to us as well"*

Date __/__/__

AM ☀ **I'm grateful for...**

1. _____
2. _____
3. _____
4. _____
5. _____

I set goals and I reach them.

PM ☾ **Things I did for myself today....**

1. _____
2. _____
3. _____
4. _____

"When you are grateful, fear disappears and abundance appears."

Date __/__/__

AM ☀ I'm grateful for...

1. _____
2. _____
3. _____
4. _____
5. _____

Today, I will walk through my fears.

PM ☾ People I'm grateful for today....

1. _____
2. _____
3. _____
4. _____

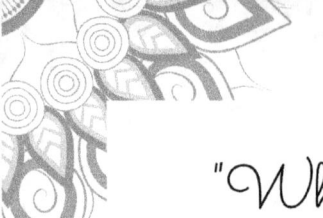

"When we give cheerfully and accept gratefully, everyone is blessed."

Date __/__/__

AM ☀ I'm grateful for...

1. _____
2. _____
3. _____
4. _____
5. _____

I am at peace with myself.

PM ☾ 3 Amazing things that happened today....

1. _____
2. _____
3. _____
4. _____

"I thank everything, because everything teaches me something.."

Date __/__/__

AM ☀ **I'm grateful for...**

1. _____
2. _____
3. _____
4. _____
5. _____

My potential to succeed is infinite.

PM ☾ **How could I have made today even better....**

1. _____
2. _____
3. _____
4. _____

"Don't pray when it rains if you don't pray when the sun shines.."

Date __/__/__

AM ☀ I'm grateful for...

1. _____
2. _____
3. _____
4. _____
5. _____

I am proud of my own success.

PM ☾ Small victories I had today....

1. _____
2. _____
3. _____
4. _____

"Acknowledging the good that you already have in your life is the foundation for all abundance."

Date __/__/__

AM ☀ I'm grateful for...

1. _____
2. _____
3. _____
4. _____
5. _____

I celebrate my individuality.

PM ☾ Things I did for myself today....

1. _____
2. _____
3. _____
4. _____

"Giving thanks for abundance is greater than the abundance itself.."

Date __/__/__

AM ☀ I'm grateful for...

1. _____
2. _____
3. _____
4. _____
5. _____

I am my own superhero.

PM ☾ People I'm grateful for today....

1. _____
2. _____
3. _____
4. _____

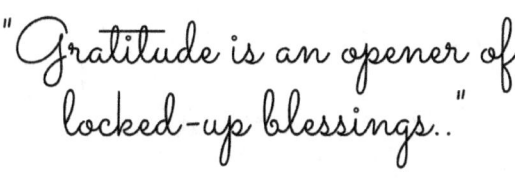

"Gratitude is an opener of locked-up blessings.."

Date _/_/_

AM ☀ I'm grateful for...

1. _____
2. _____
3. _____
4. _____
5. _____

I am free to be myself.

PM ☾ 3 Amazing things that happened today....

1. _____
2. _____
3. _____
4. _____

"When I started counting my blessings, my whole life turned around."

Date __/__/__

AM ☀ I'm grateful for...

1. _____
2. _____
3. _____
4. _____
5. _____

I trust myself.

PM ☾ How could I have made today even better....

1. _____
2. _____
3. _____
4. _____

"*Gratitude is merely the secret hope of further favors..*"

Date ___/___/___

AM ☀ **I'm grateful for...**

1. _____
2. _____
3. _____
4. _____
5. _____

I am free to be myself.

PM ☾ **Small victories I had today....**

1. _____
2. _____
3. _____
4. _____

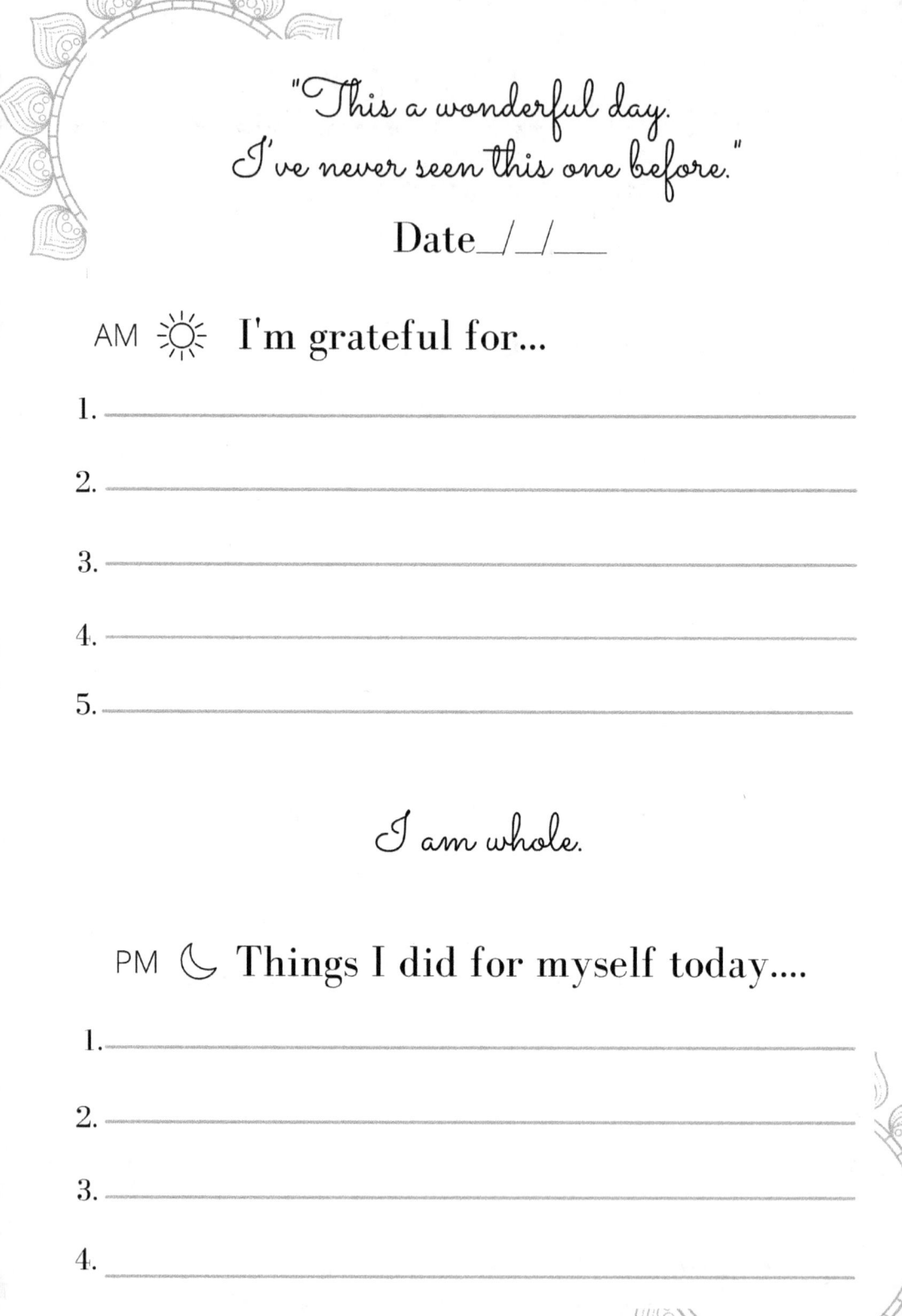

"This a wonderful day.
I've never seen this one before."

Date __/__/__

AM ☀ I'm grateful for...

1. _____
2. _____
3. _____
4. _____
5. _____

I am whole.

PM ☾ Things I did for myself today....

1. _____
2. _____
3. _____
4. _____

"The essence of all beautiful art is gratitude.."

Date __/__/__

AM ☼ I'm grateful for...

1. ___
2. ___
3. ___
4. ___
5. ___

I am enough.

PM ☾ People I'm grateful for today....

1. ___
2. ___
3. ___
4. ___

"Gratitude goes beyond the 'mine' and 'thine' and claims the truth that all of life is a pure gift."

Date __/__/__

AM ☀ **I'm grateful for...**

1. _____
2. _____
3. _____
4. _____
5. _____

My potential to succeed is infinite.

PM ☾ **3 Amazing things that happened today....**

1. _____
2. _____
3. _____
4. _____

"*Nothing is more honorable than a grateful heart.*"

Date __/__/__

AM ☀ **I'm grateful for...**

1. _____
2. _____
3. _____
4. _____
5. _____

I live each day to the fullest.

PM ☾ **How could I have made today even better....**

1. _____
2. _____
3. _____
4. _____

"Not what we say about our blessings, but how we use them, is the true measure of our thanksgiving."

Date __/__/__

AM ☀ I'm grateful for...

1. _____
2. _____
3. _____
4. _____
5. _____

I am proud of myself and all that I have accomplished.

PM ☾ Small victories I had today....

1. _____
2. _____
3. _____
4. _____

"When you are grateful, fear disappears and abundance appears"

Date __/__/__

AM ☀ **I'm grateful for...**

1. _____
2. _____
3. _____
4. _____
5. _____

I take pride in the progress I make each day.

PM ☾ **Things I did for myself today....**

1. _____
2. _____
3. _____
4. _____

"There are always flowers for those who want to see them."

Date __/__/__

AM ☀ I'm grateful for...

1. _____
2. _____
3. _____
4. _____
5. _____

People like me, and I feel good about myself.

PM ☾ People I'm grateful for today....

1. _____
2. _____
3. _____
4. _____

"Giving is an expression of gratitude for our blessings."

Date __/__/__

AM ☀ **I'm grateful for...**

1. _____
2. _____
3. _____
4. _____
5. _____

I respect and treat myself with kindness and love.

PM ☾ **3 Amazing things that happened today....**

1. _____
2. _____
3. _____
4. _____

"*An attitude of gratitude brings great things.*"

Date __/__/__

AM ☀ I'm grateful for...

1. _____
2. _____
3. _____
4. _____
5. _____

I go for goals with passion and pride.

PM ☾ How could I have made today even better....

1. _____
2. _____
3. _____
4. _____

"Find the good and praise it."

Date __/__/__

AM ☀ **I'm grateful for...**

1. _____
2. _____
3. _____
4. _____
5. _____

The world is a better place with me in it.

PM ☾ **Small victories I had today....**

1. _____
2. _____
3. _____
4. _____

"Things must be felt with the heart."

Date _/_/_

AM ☀ I'm grateful for...

1. _____
2. _____
3. _____
4. _____
5. _____

I am worthy of greatness.

PM ☾ Things I did for myself today....

1. _____
2. _____
3. _____
4. _____

"Appreciation is the purest vibration that exists on the planet today."

Date __/__/__

AM ☀ I'm grateful for...

1. _____
2. _____
3. _____
4. _____
5. _____

I am never a burden.

PM ☾ People I'm grateful for today....

1. _____
2. _____
3. _____
4. _____

"May the gratitude in your heart kiss all the universe."

Date __/__/__

AM ☀ I'm grateful for...

1. _____
2. _____
3. _____
4. _____
5. _____

I am at peace with myself.

PM ☾ 3 Amazing things that happened today....

1. _____
2. _____
3. _____
4. _____

"Gratitude unlocks the fullness of life."

Date __/__/__

☀ **AM** **I'm grateful for...**

1. _____

2. _____

3. _____

4. _____

5. _____

I am smart, capable and valuable.

🌙 **PM** **How could I have made today even better....**

1. _____

2. _____

3. _____

4. _____

"When we give cheerfully and accept gratefully, everyone is blessed."

Date __/__/__

AM ☀ I'm grateful for...

1. ___
2. ___
3. ___
4. ___
5. ___

I am unique in my own wonderful way.

PM ☾ Small victories I had today....

1. ___
2. ___
3. ___
4. ___

"The trick is to be grateful when your mood is high and graceful when it is low."

Date __/__/__

AM ☀ **I'm grateful for...**

1. _____

2. _____

3. _____

4. _____

5. _____

I accept myself as I am.

PM ☾ **Things I did for myself today....**

1. _____

2. _____

3. _____

4. _____

"Do not spoil what you have by desiring what you have not."

Date __/__/__

AM ☀ I'm grateful for...

1. _____
2. _____
3. _____
4. _____
5. _____

I am focused, persistent and will never quit.

PM ☾ People I'm grateful for today....

1. _____
2. _____
3. _____
4. _____

*"The more grateful I am,
the more beauty I see."*

Date __/__/__

AM ☀ **I'm grateful for...**

1. _____
2. _____
3. _____
4. _____
5. _____

I accept myself as I am.

PM ☾ **3 Amazing things that happened today....**

1. _____
2. _____
3. _____
4. _____

"Be grateful, not only for others, but for yourself"

Date __/__/__

AM ☀ I'm grateful for...

1. _____
2. _____
3. _____
4. _____
5. _____

I have the power to create change.

PM ☾ How could I have made today even better....

1. _____
2. _____
3. _____
4. _____

"A grateful mind is a great mind which eventually attracts to itself great things."

Date __/__/__

AM ☀ I'm grateful for...

1. _____
2. _____
3. _____
4. _____
5. _____

I am in charge of my own happiness.

PM ☾ Small victories I had today....

1. _____
2. _____
3. _____
4. _____

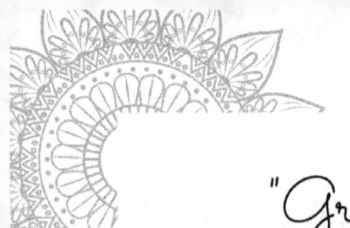

"Gratitude changes the pangs of memory into a tranquil joy."

Date __/__/__

AM ☀ I'm grateful for...

1. _____
2. _____
3. _____
4. _____
5. _____

I have courage and confidence.

PM ☾ Things I did for myself today....

1. _____
2. _____
3. _____
4. _____

"Expressing gratitude is a natural state of being and reminds us that we are all connected.."

Date __/__/__

AM ☼ **I'm grateful for...**

1. _____
2. _____
3. _____
4. _____
5. _____

I take pride in my achievements.

PM ☾ **People I'm grateful for today....**

1. _____
2. _____
3. _____
4. _____

"Now is no time to think of what you do not have. Think of what you can do with what there is."

Date __/__/__

AM ☀ I'm grateful for...

1. _____
2. _____
3. _____
4. _____
5. _____

I don't need to be perfect.

PM ☾ 3 Amazing things that happened today....

1. _____
2. _____
3. _____
4. _____

"Gratitude for the present moment and the fullness of life now is the true prosperity."

Date __/__/__

AM ☀ **I'm grateful for...**

1. _____
2. _____
3. _____
4. _____
5. _____

I can get through anything.

PM ☾ **How could I have made today even better....**

1. _____
2. _____
3. _____
4. _____

"When it comes to life the critical thing is whether you take things for granted or take them with gratitude"

Date __/__/__

AM ☀ **I'm grateful for...**

1. _____
2. _____
3. _____
4. _____
5. _____

I love myself.

PM ☾ **Small victories I had today....**

1. _____
2. _____
3. _____
4. _____

"Breathe. Let go. And remind yourself that this very moment is the only one you know you have for sure"

Date __/__/__

AM ☀ **I'm grateful for...**

1. _____
2. _____
3. _____
4. _____
5. _____

I am an amazing person.

PM ☾ **Things I did for myself today....**

1. _____
2. _____
3. _____
4. _____

"There is a calmness to a life lived in gratitude, a quiet joy"

Date __/__/__

AM ☀ I'm grateful for...

1. _____
2. _____
3. _____
4. _____
5. _____

I can make a difference.

PM ☾ People I'm grateful for today....

1. _____
2. _____
3. _____
4. _____

*"You cannot do a kindness too soon
because you never know how soon
it will be too late."*

Date __/__/__

AM ☀ **I'm grateful for...**

1. _____
2. _____
3. _____
4. _____
5. _____

I can do anything.

PM ☾ **3 Amazing things that happened today....**

1. _____
2. _____
3. _____
4. _____

"You don't get blessed, and feel blessed. You have to first feel blessed, then the blessings come to you.."

Date __/__/__

AM ☀ I'm grateful for...

1. _____
2. _____
3. _____
4. _____
5. _____

I set goals and I reach them.

PM ☾ How could I have made today even better....

1. _____
2. _____
3. _____
4. _____

"The thankful receiver bears a plentiful harvest."

Date __/__/__

AM ☀ **I'm grateful for...**

1. _____
2. _____
3. _____
4. _____
5. _____

I am in charge of my life.

PM ☾ **Small victories I had today....**

1. _____
2. _____
3. _____
4. _____

"Among the things you can give and still keep are your word, a smile, and a grateful heart.."

Date __/__/__

AM ☀ I'm grateful for...

1. _____
2. _____
3. _____
4. _____
5. _____

I am at peace with myself.

PM ☾ Things I did for myself today....

1. _____
2. _____
3. _____
4. _____

> *"There's no disaster that can't become a blessing, and no blessing that can't become a disaster.."*

Date __/__/__

AM ☀ I'm grateful for...

1. _____
2. _____
3. _____
4. _____
5. _____

Today, I will walk through my fears.

PM ☾ People I'm grateful for today....

1. _____
2. _____
3. _____
4. _____

"Train yourself never to put off the word or action for the expression of gratitude.."

Date _/_/__

AM ☼ I'm grateful for...

1. _____
2. _____
3. _____
4. _____
5. _____

I am proud of my own success.

PM ☾ 3 Amazing things that happened today....

1. _____
2. _____
3. _____
4. _____

"There's no happier person than a truly thankful, content person."

Date __/__/__

AM ☀ I'm grateful for...

1. _____
2. _____
3. _____
4. _____
5. _____

My potential to succeed is infinite.

PM ☾ How could I have made today even better....

1. _____
2. _____
3. _____
4. _____

"Opening your eyes to more of the world around you can deeply enhance your gratitude practice"

Date __/__/__

AM ☀ I'm grateful for...

1. _____
2. _____
3. _____
4. _____
5. _____

I am my own superhero.

PM ☾ Small victories I had today....

1. _____
2. _____
3. _____
4. _____

*"Gratitude is the wine for the soul.
Go on. Get drunk.."*

Date __/__/__

AM ☀ I'm grateful for...

1. _____
2. _____
3. _____
4. _____
5. _____

I celebrate my individuality.

PM ☾ Things I did for myself today....

1. _____
2. _____
3. _____
4. _____

"Gratitude can turn a meal into a feast."

Date __/__/__

AM ☼ **I'm grateful for...**

1. _____
2. _____
3. _____
4. _____
5. _____

I trust myself.

PM ☾ **People I'm grateful for today....**

1. _____
2. _____
3. _____
4. _____

"The hardest arithmetic to master is that which enables us to count our blessings."

Date __/__/__

AM ☀ **I'm grateful for...**

1. _____
2. _____
3. _____
4. _____
5. _____

I am free to be myself.

PM ☾ **3 Amazing things that happened today....**

1. _____
2. _____
3. _____
4. _____

"Let us live simply in the freshness of the present moment, in the clarity of pure awakened mind.."

Date __/__/__

AM ☀ **I'm grateful for...**

1. _____
2. _____
3. _____
4. _____
5. _____

I am whole.

PM ☾ **How could I have made today even better....**

1. _____
2. _____
3. _____
4. _____

"When you have something use it with appreciation before you lose it and always remember those who don't have it."

Date ___/___/___

AM ☀ I'm grateful for...

1. _____
2. _____
3. _____
4. _____
5. _____

I am free to be myself.

PM ☾ Small victories I had today....

1. _____
2. _____
3. _____
4. _____

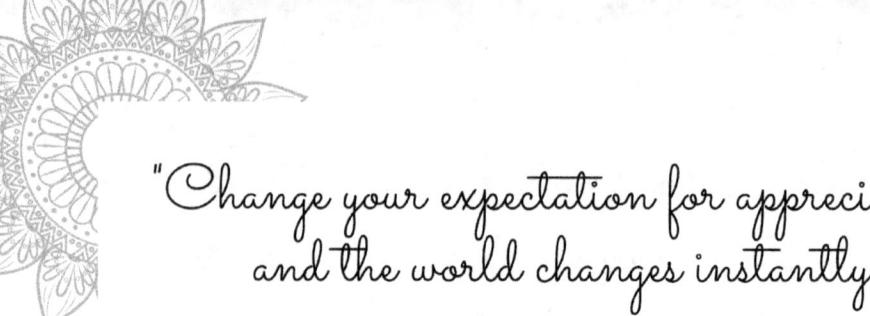

"Change your expectation for appreciation and the world changes instantly"

Date __/__/__

AM ☀ **I'm grateful for...**

1. _____
2. _____
3. _____
4. _____
5. _____

My potential to succeed is infinite.

PM ☾ **Things I did for myself today....**

1. _____
2. _____
3. _____
4. _____

"While it may be difficult to change the world, it is always possible to change the way we look at it.."

Date __/__/__

AM ☀ I'm grateful for...

1. _____
2. _____
3. _____
4. _____
5. _____

I live each day to the fullest.

PM ☾ People I'm grateful for today....

1. _____
2. _____
3. _____
4. _____

"Wisdom and compassion should become the dominating influences that guide our thoughts, our words, and our actions."

Date __/__/__

AM ☀ I'm grateful for...

1. _____
2. _____
3. _____
4. _____
5. _____

I am proud of myself and all that I have accomplished.

PM ☾ 3 Amazing things that happened today....

1. _____
2. _____
3. _____
4. _____

"Love those who appreciate you, and appreciate those who love you.."

Date __/__/__

AM ☀ I'm grateful for...

1. _____
2. _____
3. _____
4. _____
5. _____

I live each day to the fullest.

PM ☾ How could I have made today even better....

1. _____
2. _____
3. _____
4. _____

"Yesterday is history. Tomorrow is a mystery but today is a gift. That's why they call it the present."

Date __/__/__

AM ☼ I'm grateful for...

1. _____
2. _____
3. _____
4. _____
5. _____

I am proud of myself and all that I have accomplished.

PM ☾ Small victories I had today....

1. _____
2. _____
3. _____
4. _____

"The struggle ends when gratitude begins."
Date __/__/__

AM ☼ I'm grateful for...

1. ___
2. ___
3. ___
4. ___
5. ___

I take pride in the progress I make each day.

PM ☾ Things I did for myself today....

1. ___
2. ___
3. ___
4. ___

"The roots of all goodness lie in the soil of appreciation for goodness."

Date __/__/__

AM ☼ I'm grateful for...

1. _____
2. _____
3. _____
4. _____
5. _____

People like me, and I feel good about myself.

PM ☾ People I'm grateful for today....

1. _____
2. _____
3. _____
4. _____

"The best way to pay for a lovely moment is to enjoy it.."

Date __/__/__

AM ☀ **I'm grateful for...**

1. _____
2. _____
3. _____
4. _____
5. _____

I respect and treat myself with kindness and love.

PM ☾ **3 Amazing things that happened today....**

1. _____
2. _____
3. _____
4. _____

"Strive to find things to be thankful for, and just look for the good in who you are."

Date __/__/__

AM ☀ I'm grateful for...

1. _____
2. _____
3. _____
4. _____
5. _____

I go for goals with passion and pride.

PM ☾ How could I have made today even better....

1. _____
2. _____
3. _____
4. _____

"You won't be happy with more until you're happy with what you've got.."

Date __/__/__

AM ☀ I'm grateful for...

1. _____
2. _____
3. _____
4. _____
5. _____

The world is a better place with me in it.

PM ☾ Small victories I had today....

1. _____
2. _____
3. _____
4. _____

"If you do not appreciate every day of your life, who said that the days and years will be an asset for the future?"

Date __/__/__

AM ☀ **I'm grateful for...**

1. _____
2. _____
3. _____
4. _____
5. _____

I am worthy of greatness.

PM ☾ **Things I did for myself today....**

1. _____
2. _____
3. _____
4. _____

"It is not happy people who are thankful, it is thankful people who are happy."

Date __/__/__

AM ☀ I'm grateful for...

1. _____
2. _____
3. _____
4. _____
5. _____

I am never a burden.

PM ☾ People I'm grateful for today....

1. _____
2. _____
3. _____
4. _____

"God gave you a gift of 86,400 seconds today. Have you used one to say "thank you?"

Date __/__/__

AM ☀ I'm grateful for...

1. ___
2. ___
3. ___
4. ___
5. ___

I am smart, capable and valuable.

PM ☾ 3 Amazing things that happened today....

1. ___
2. ___
3. ___
4. ___

"The way to develop the best that is in a person is by appreciation and encouragement."

Date __/__/__

AM ☀ **I'm grateful for...**

1. _____
2. _____
3. _____
4. _____
5. _____

I am unique in my own wonderful way.

PM ☾ **How could I have made today even better....**

1. _____
2. _____
3. _____
4. _____

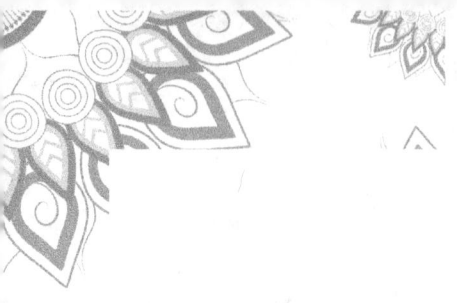

Copyrights 2021 - All rights reserved

You may not reproduce, duplicate, or send the contents of this book without direct written permission from the author. You cannot hereby despite any circumstance blame the publisher or hold him or her the legal responsibility for any reparation, compensation or monetary forfeiture owing to the information included herein, either in a direct or indirect way.

Legal Notice: This book has copyright protection. You can use the book for personal purpose. You should not sell, use, alter, distribute, quote, take excerpts or paraphrase in part of whole the material contained in this book without obtaining the permission of the author first.

Disclaimer Notice: You must take note that the information in this document is for casual reading and entertainment purpose only. We have made every attempt to provide accurate, up to date and reliable information. We do not express or imply guarantees of any kind. The person who read admit that the writer is not occupied in giving legal, financial, medical, or other advice. We put this book content by sourcing various places.

Please consult a licensed professional before you try any techniques shown in this book. By going through this document, the book lover comes to an agreement that under no situation is the author accountable for any forfeiture, direct or indirect, which they may incur because of the use of material contained in this document, including, but not limited to, - errors, omissions, or inaccuracies.

CREATEPUBLICATION

Thank you!

As a small family company, your feedback is very important to us.

Please let us know how you like our book at:

/createpublication

/createpublication

createpublication@gmail.com

www.ingramcontent.com/pod-product-compliance
Lightning Source LLC
Chambersburg PA
CBHW071502070526
44578CB00001B/418